INTRODUCTION

Welcome to the invigorating and tasty universe of detox recipes!

This book is more than a cooking guide; It is an invitation to transform your diet in a healthy and delicious way. Here, we will dive together into a world of fresh ingredients, balanced combinations and dishes that not only nourish your body, but also provide an unparalleled gastronomic experience.

Throughout the pages, you will find a variety of carefully selected recipes to boost your health and well-being. Each dish is made with ingredients that detoxify the body, promote vitality and offer an explosion of flavors that stimulate the senses. From revitalizing juices to comforting soups and nutrient-packed salads, our goal is to provide you with a diverse menu that will make the detox process an experience.

pleasurable.

To ensure you get the most out of each recipe, we rely on the expertise of professionals who share valuable tips throughout the book. These experts not only guide you through step-by-step preparation, but also offer insights into the best way to serve each dish, ensuring a complete dining experience.

We believe that healthy eating does not have to be monotonous; on the contrary, it can be an exciting and delicious journey. By following the recipes in this book, you will not only take care of your body, but also allow yourself to enjoy balanced and delicious cuisine. We look forward to guiding you on this culinary journey, where each recipe is more than a dish – it's a step towards a healthier, more vibrant life. Get ready to savor the balance and vitality in every bite and sip.

"Enjoy an invigorating culinary experience with our detox cookbook! Each recipe is a celebration of fresh, nutritious flavors designed to revitalize your body. Allow yourself to savor the best of health and gastronomic pleasure as you embark on this delicious and detoxifying journey."

<u>SUMMARY</u>

DETOX SALADS

Detox Green Salad

Colorful Detox Salad

Detox Quinoa Salad

Detox Fruit Salad

Detox Lentil Salad

Detox Cucumber Salad

Detox Avocado Salad

Detox Kale Salad

Detox Pear Salad

Detox Broccoli Salad

Detox Watermelon Salad

Detox Seaweed Salad

Detox Bean Salad

Detox Zucchini Salad

Detox Strawberry Salad

Detox Pumpkin Salad

Detox Mushroom Salad

Detox Asparagus Salad

DETOX SOUPS

Detox green broth with kale

Carrot and celery soup

Creamed spinach with leeks

Lentil soup with vegetables

Roasted tomato soup with basil

Cauliflower cream with turmeric

Beetroot soup with mint

Chickpea soup with spinach

Vegetable broth with quinoa

Zucchini soup with cilantro

Asparagus cream with lemon

Broccoli soup with saffron

Leek soup with sweet potato

Mushroom soup with rosemary

Green lentil broth with turmeric

Tomato and red pepper soup

Kale soup with chia

Asparagus cream with basil

Green Detox Juice

Ingredients:

• 1 green apple, peeled and chopped • 1 medium
cucumber, peeled and cut into slices • 1 handful of fresh spinach •
1/2 lemon, juiced • 1 teaspoon of grated
ginger • 1 glass of coconut
water • Ice cubes (optional)

Method of preparation:

1. **Preparation of Ingredients:** • Peel and
   chop the green apple. • Peel and cut the
   cucumber into slices. • Squeeze the juice from half a
   lemon. • Grate the ginger to get a teaspoon.

2. **Juice Assembly:**
   • In a blender, add the green apple, cucumber, spinach, lemon juice
   lemon and grated ginger.

3. **Addition of Liquids:**
   • Pour the glass of coconut water over the ingredients in the blender.

4. **Beat Well:**
   • Beat all ingredients until you obtain a homogeneous and smooth mixture.

5. **Straining (Optional):**
   • If you prefer a finer texture, strain the juice using a fine strainer.

6. **Adding Ice (Optional):** • Add ice
   cubes to the juice if you want a colder drink.

7. **Serve Immediately:**
   • Pour the green detox juice into a glass and serve immediately to make the most of the benefits of the
   fresh ingredients.

Tip: If desired, decorate the glass with a thin slice of cucumber or a mint leaf for a visually attractive
touch.

This green detox juice is rich in nutrients, antioxidants and fiber, providing a refreshing and healthy drink
to incorporate into your detox routine.

Energizing Juice

Ingredients:

• 1 carrot, peeled and cut into pieces • 1 orange, peeled and
divided into wedges • 1/2 beetroot, peeled and chopped •
1 apple, peeled and chopped • 1 teaspoon of
honey • 1 glass of water • Cubes of ice
(optional)

Method of preparation:

1. **Preparation of Ingredients:** • Peel and
cut the carrot into pieces. • Peel the orange and separate
it into segments. • Peel and chop the beetroot. • Remove
the skin from the apple and cut into pieces.

2. **Assembling the Juice:** •
Place the carrot, orange, beetroot and apple in the blender.
3. **Addition of Honey:**
• Add a teaspoon of honey to the ingredients in the blender.
4. **Addition of Liquids:**
• Pour a glass of water over the ingredients.
5. **Beat Well:**
• Beat all ingredients until you obtain a smooth and homogeneous mixture.
6. **Adding Ice (Optional):** • If desired,
add ice cubes for a colder texture.
7. **Serve Immediately:**
• Pour the energizing juice into a glass and serve immediately.

Tip: Garnish the glass with a thin slice of orange or a mint leaf for a visually appealing touch. This
energizing juice is a great option to start the day with vitality and promote an invigorating feeling.

Beetroot Detox Juice

Ingredients:

• 1 medium beet, peeled and cut into cubes • 1 green
apple, peeled and chopped • 1 carrot,
peeled and cut into slices • 1/2 lemon, juiced • 1
teaspoon of grated ginger
• 1 glass of water • Cubes ice (optional)

Method of preparation:

1. **Preparation of Ingredients:** •
   Peel and cut the beetroot into cubes. • Remove
   the skin from the green apple and chop it. •
   Peel and cut the carrot into slices. • Squeeze
   the juice from half a lemon. • Grate
   the ginger to get a teaspoon.
2. **Juice Assembly:**
   • Place the beetroot, green apple, carrot, lemon juice and ginger in the
   blender.
3. **Adding Liquids:** •
   Pour a glass of water over the ingredients in the blender.
4. **Beat Well:**
   • Beat all ingredients until you obtain a smooth and homogeneous mixture.
5. **Adding Ice (Optional):** • If
   desired, add ice cubes for a colder texture.
6. **Serve Immediately:**
   • Pour the beetroot detox juice into a glass and serve immediately.

Tip: Garnish the glass with some thin beetroot slices for a visually appealing
touch. This beetroot detox juice is an excellent choice for detoxification, providing
essential nutrients and a vibrant flavor.

Antioxidant Juice

Ingredients:

• 1 cup fresh blueberries

• 1 cup of strawberries, without leaves • 1
orange, peeled and divided into wedges • 1/2 cucumber,
peeled and cut into slices • 1 teaspoon of chia seeds (optional)

• 1 cup of coconut water • Cubes of ice (optional)

Method of preparation:

1. **Preparation of Ingredients:** • Wash
the blueberries and strawberries well. • Remove
the leaves from the strawberries. • Peel the
orange and separate it into segments. • Peel and cut
the cucumber into slices.

2. **Juice Assembly:**
• Add blueberries, strawberries, orange, cucumber and chia seeds (if available).
using) in the blender.

3. **Addition of Liquids:**
• Pour the glass of coconut water over the ingredients in the blender.

4. **Beat Well:**
• Beat all ingredients until you obtain a smooth and homogeneous mixture.

5. **Adding Ice (Optional):** • If you
prefer, add ice cubes for a refreshing touch.

6. **Serve Immediately:**
• Pour the antioxidant juice into a glass and serve immediately.

Tip: Garnish the glass with some blueberries or thin orange slices for a visually appealing touch. This
antioxidant juice is rich in natural antioxidants, helping to fight free radicals and promote cellular
health.

Refreshing Watermelon Juice

Ingredients:

• 2 cups watermelon, seeded and diced • 1/2 cucumber, peeled and cut into
pieces • 1 lemon, juiced • 1 teaspoon fresh mint, chopped • 1
teaspoon grated ginger • 1
cup water • Ice cubes (optional)

Method of preparation:

1. **Preparation of Ingredients:** • Cut the
watermelon into cubes, removing the seeds. • Peel and cut the cucumber
into pieces. • Squeeze the lemon juice. • Finely chop the
fresh mint. • Grate the ginger to get
a teaspoon.

2. **Juice Assembly:**
• Place the watermelon, cucumber, lemon juice, mint and ginger cubes in the
blender.
3. **Adding Liquids:** • Pour
the glass of water over the ingredients in the blender.
4. **Beat Well:**
• Beat all ingredients until you obtain a smooth and homogeneous mixture.
5. **Adding Ice (Optional):** • If you
prefer, add ice cubes for a more refreshing experience.
6. **Serve Immediately:**
• Pour the refreshing watermelon juice into a glass and serve immediately.

Tip: Garnish the glass with a thin slice of watermelon or a mint leaf for a visually appealing touch. This
refreshing juice is a hydrating and delicious option for hot days.

Pineapple Detox Juice

Ingredients:

• 1 cup fresh pineapple, diced • 1 cucumber , peeled and
sliced • 1 apple, peeled and chopped • 1 lemon, juiced • 1
teaspoon grated ginger • 1 handful of
mint leaves • 1 cup of water
• Ice cubes (optional)

Method of preparation:

1. Preparation of Ingredients:
• Cut the pineapple into cubes. • Peel
and cut the cucumber into slices. • Chop the apple,
removing the skin. • Squeeze the lemon juice.
• Grate the ginger to get a teaspoon.
• Wash and dry the mint leaves.

2. Juice Assembly:
• Place the pineapple, cucumber, apple, lemon juice, ginger and mint leaves in a blender.

3. **Adding Liquids:** • Pour
the glass of water over the ingredients in the blender.

4. Beat Well:
• Beat all ingredients until you obtain a smooth and homogeneous mixture.

5. **Adding Ice (Optional):** • If you
prefer, add ice cubes for a colder texture.

6. **Serve Immediately:** • Pour
the pineapple detox juice into a glass and serve immediately.

Tip: Decorate the glass with a slice of cucumber or a mint leaf for a visually appealing touch. This
pineapple detox juice is a delicious option full of nutrients to promote detoxification of the body.

Pear Digestive Juice

Ingredients:

• 2 ripe pears, peeled and cut into pieces • 1 kiwi, peeled and cut into
pieces • 1/2 pineapple, peeled and cut into cubes • 1
teaspoon fresh mint, chopped • 1 teaspoon flax seeds
(optional) • 1 glass of water • Ice cubes (optional)

Method of preparation:

1. **Preparation of Ingredients:** • Peel and
cut the pears into pieces. • Peel and cut the kiwi into
pieces. • Cut the pineapple into cubes. • Finely chop
the mint.

2. **Juice Assembly:**
• Add pears, kiwi, pineapple, mint and flaxseeds (if available).
using) in the blender.

3. **Adding Liquids:** • Pour
the glass of water over the ingredients in the blender.

4. **Beat Well:**
• Beat all ingredients until you obtain a smooth and homogeneous mixture.

5. **Adding Ice (Optional):** • If you
prefer, add ice cubes for a more refreshing experience.

6. **Serve Immediately:**
• Pour the pear digestive juice into a glass and serve immediately.

Tip: Garnish the glass with a thin slice of kiwi or a few mint leaves for a visually appealing touch. This pear
digestive juice is a great option to promote digestion and provide essential nutrients in a delicious way.

Kale and Pineapple Detox Juice

Ingredients:

• 2 kale leaves, without the central stem • 1 cup of
pineapple, cut into pieces • 1 green apple, peeled and
chopped • 1 lemon, juiced • 1 teaspoon of
grated ginger • 1 cup of
coconut water • Cubes ice (optional)

Method of preparation:

1. Preparation of Ingredients:
  • Remove the central stalk from the cabbage leaves.
  • Cut the pineapple into pieces. • Chop
  the green apple. • Squeeze
  the lemon juice. • Grate the ginger
  to get a teaspoon.

2. Juice Assembly:
  • Add cabbage leaves, pineapple, green apple, lemon juice and ginger
    grated in a blender.

3. Addition of Liquids:
  • Pour the glass of coconut water over the ingredients in the blender.

4. Beat Well:
  • Beat all ingredients until you obtain a smooth and homogeneous mixture.

5. Adding Ice (Optional): • If you
  prefer, add ice cubes for a colder texture.

6. Serve Immediately:
  • Pour the kale and pineapple detox juice into a glass and serve immediately.

Tip: Garnish the glass with a thin slice of pineapple or a kale leaf for a visually appealing touch. This
detox juice is an excellent choice for detoxification and supplying essential nutrients.

Purifying Apple Juice

Ingredients:

• 2 red apples, peeled and cut into slices • 1 carrot, peeled and cut into slices • 1/2 cucumber, peeled and cut into pieces • 1 teaspoon grated ginger • 1 teaspoon lemon juice • 1 cup of water • Ice cubes (optional)

Method of preparation:

1. **Preparation of Ingredients:** • Peel and cut the apples into slices. • Peel and cut the carrot into slices. • Peel and cut the cucumber into pieces. • Grate the ginger to get a teaspoon.

2. **Juice Assembly:**
   • Place the apples, carrots, cucumber, ginger and lemon juice in a blender.

3. **Adding Liquids:** • Pour the glass of water over the ingredients in the blender.

4. **Beat Well:**
   • Beat all ingredients until you obtain a smooth and homogeneous mixture.

5. **Adding Ice (Optional):** • If you prefer, add ice cubes for a colder texture.

6. **Serve Immediately:**
   • Pour the purifying apple juice into a glass and serve immediately.

Tip: Garnish the glass with a thin slice of apple or a slice of cucumber for a visually appealing touch. This purifying apple juice is an excellent option for cleansing the body and enjoying a naturally sweet flavor.

Eggplant Detox Juice

Ingredients:

• 1 medium eggplant, cut into cubes • 1 green
apple, peeled and chopped • 1 lemon, juiced •
1 teaspoon fresh mint,
chopped • 1 teaspoon chia seeds (optional) • 1 glass of
water • Ice cubes (optional)

Method of preparation:

1. **Preparation of Ingredients:** • Cut the
eggplant into cubes. • Chop the green
apple. • Squeeze the lemon
juice. • Finely chop the mint.

2. **Juice Assembly:**
• Place the eggplant, green apple, lemon juice, mint and chia seeds (if using) in a blender.

3. **Adding Liquids:** • Pour
the glass of water over the ingredients in the blender.

4. **Beat Well:**
• Beat all ingredients until you obtain a smooth and homogeneous mixture.

5. **Adding Ice (Optional):** • If you
prefer, add ice cubes for a colder texture.

6. **Serve Immediately:**
• Pour the eggplant detox juice into a glass and serve immediately.

Tip: Decorate the glass with a mint leaf or some chia seeds for a visually appealing touch. This eggplant detox juice is a nutritious and tasty option to include in your detox routine.

Revitalizing Red Fruit Juice

Ingredients:

• 1 cup strawberries, leafless • 1/2 cup
raspberries • 1/2 cup blueberries • 1
red apple, peeled and chopped
• 1 teaspoon honey • 1 teaspoon lemon juice

• 1 glass of water • Ice
cubes (optional)

Method of preparation:

1. **Preparation of Ingredients:** • Remove
   the leaves from the strawberries. • Wash
   strawberries, raspberries and blueberries well. • Chop the red
   apple. • Squeeze the lemon juice.

2. **Juice Assembly:**
   • Place the strawberries, raspberries, blueberries, red apple, honey and lemon juice in the blender.

3. **Adding Liquids:** • Pour
   the glass of water over the ingredients in the blender.

4. **Beat Well:**
   • Beat all ingredients until you obtain a smooth and homogeneous mixture.

5. **Adding Ice (Optional):** • If you
   prefer, add ice cubes for a more refreshing experience.

6. **Serve Immediately:**
   • Pour the revitalizing red fruit juice into a glass and serve
   immediately.

Tip: Garnish the glass with some whole strawberries or raspberries for a visually appealing touch. This
revitalizing juice is rich in antioxidants and vitamins, providing a burst of refreshing flavor.

Anti-Cellulite juice

Ingredients:

• 1 cup pineapple, cut into pieces • 1/2 cucumber,
peeled and cut into slices • 1 green apple, peeled and chopped
• 1/2 lemon, juiced • 1 teaspoon grated ginger
• 1 teaspoon fresh mint,
chopped • 1 cup green tea, chilled • Ice cubes
(optional)

Method of preparation:

1. **Preparation of Ingredients:** • Cut the
    pineapple into pieces. • Peel and cut the
    cucumber into slices. • Chop the green apple. •
    Squeeze the juice from half a
    lemon. • Grate the ginger to get a teaspoon.
    • Finely chop the mint.

2. **Juice Assembly:**
    • Place pineapple, cucumber, green apple, lemon juice, ginger and mint in the
        blender.

3. **Addition of Liquids:**
    • Pour the cooled glass of green tea over the ingredients in the blender.

4. **Beat Well:**
    • Beat all ingredients until you obtain a smooth and homogeneous mixture.

5. **Adding Ice (Optional):** • If you
    prefer, add ice cubes for a colder texture.

6. **Serve Immediately:**
    • Pour the anti-cellulite juice into a glass and serve immediately.

Tip: Garnish the glass with a thin slice of cucumber or a mint leaf for a visually appealing touch. This anti-cellulite juice is a refreshing option that combines ingredients known for their potential benefits for skin health.

Melon Detox Juice

Ingredients:

• 2 cups of melon, cut into cubes • 1 orange, peeled
and divided into wedges • 1 carrot, peeled and cut into
slices • 1 teaspoon of grated ginger • 1 teaspoon of honey •
1 glass of water • Cubes of ice (optional)

Method of preparation:

1. Preparation of Ingredients:
> • Cut the melon into cubes.

> • Peel the orange and separate it into segments. • Peel
and cut the carrot into slices. • Grate the ginger to get a
teaspoon.

2. Juice Assembly:
> • Place the melon cubes, orange segments, carrots, ginger and honey in the
> blender.

3. Adding Liquids: • Pour
the glass of water over the ingredients in the blender.

4. Beat Well:
> • Beat all ingredients until you obtain a smooth and homogeneous mixture.

5. Adding Ice (Optional): • If you
prefer, add ice cubes for a more refreshing experience.

6. Serve Immediately:
> • Pour the melon detox juice into a glass and serve immediately.

Tip: Garnish the glass with a thin slice of orange or a few cubes of melon for a visually appealing touch.
This melon detox juice is a hydrating, vitamin-packed option to boost overall health.

Desinchá Juice

Ingredients:

• 1 teaspoon of green tea (loose leaf or sachet) • 1 cucumber, peeled and cut into wedges • 1 lemon, peeled and cut into pieces • 1 teaspoon of fresh mint, chopped • 1 teaspoon of grated ginger • 1 teaspoon of honey

• 1 glass of hot water (to prepare tea) • Ice cubes (optional)

Method of preparation:

1. Tea Preparation:

• Make an infusion of green tea, using loose leaves or a sachet, in a cup of hot water. Let the tea steep for about 5 minutes. Then let it cool.

2. Preparation of Ingredients: • Peel and cut the cucumber into slices. • Peel the lemon and cut into pieces. • Finely chop the mint. • Grate the ginger to get a teaspoon.

3. Juice Assembly:

• Place the cucumber slices, lemon pieces, mint, grated ginger and honey in the blender.

4. Addition of Liquids:

• Add the prepared green tea to the blender.

5. Beat Well:

• Beat all ingredients until you obtain a smooth and homogeneous mixture.

6. Adding Ice (Optional): • If you prefer, add ice cubes for a more refreshing experience.

7. Serve Immediately:

• Pour the deflated juice into a glass and serve immediately.

Tip: Garnish the glass with a thin slice of lemon or a mint leaf for a visually appealing touch. This desinchá juice combines ingredients known for their properties that help reduce fluid retention.

Relaxing Passion Fruit Juice

Ingredients:

• 2 passion fruits, pulp and seeds • 1 ripe
banana • 1 apple, peeled
and chopped • 1 teaspoon of honey • 1
teaspoon of dried chamomile (or
1 chamomile tea bag) • 1 glass of warm water (to prepare chamomile tea) • Ice cubes
(optional)

Method of preparation:

1. **Preparation of Chamomile Tea:** •
     Make a chamomile infusion, using loose dried flowers or a sachet,
         in a cup of warm water. Let the tea steep for about 5 minutes.
         Then let it cool.
2. **Preparation of Ingredients:** •
     Cut the passion fruit in half and remove the pulp with the seeds. •
     Peel the banana and cut into pieces. • Chop
     the apple.
3. **Juice Assembly:**
     • Place passion fruit pulp, banana, apple, honey and chamomile tea in the
         blender.
4. **Adding Liquids:** •
     Add the prepared chamomile tea to the blender.
5. **Beat Well:**
     • Beat all ingredients until you obtain a smooth and homogeneous mixture.
6. **Adding Ice (Optional):** • If
     you prefer, add ice cubes for a colder texture.
7. **Serve Immediately:**
     • Pour the relaxing passion fruit juice into a glass and serve immediately.

Tip: Decorate the glass with a thin slice of passion fruit or a mint leaf for a visually
appealing touch. This relaxing juice is perfect for moments of tranquility and
relaxation.

Avocado Detox Juice

Ingredients:

• 1 ripe avocado, peeled and pitted • 1/2 green apple, peeled
and chopped • 1 kiwi, peeled and cut into pieces
• 1 teaspoon of honey

• 1 handful of fresh spinach • 1 glass of
coconut water • Ice cubes (optional)

Method of preparation:

1. **Preparation of Ingredients:** • Peel and
remove the stone from the avocado. • Chop the green
apple. • Peel and cut the kiwi
into pieces. • Finely chop the spinach.

2. **Juice Assembly:**
• Place the avocado, green apple, kiwi, honey and spinach in the blender.

3. **Addition of Liquids:**
• Pour the glass of coconut water over the ingredients in the blender.

4. **Beat Well:**
• Beat all ingredients until you obtain a smooth and homogeneous mixture.

5. **Adding Ice (Optional):** • If you
prefer, add ice cubes for a colder texture.

6. **Serve Immediately:**
• Pour the avocado detox juice into a glass and serve immediately.

Tip: Garnish the glass with a thin slice of kiwi or a few spinach leaves for a visually appealing touch. This
avocado detox juice is a creamy and nutritious option, rich in healthy fats and vitamins.

Cucumber and Lemon Detox Juice

Ingredients:

• 1 cucumber, peeled and cut into wedges • 2 lemons,
juiced • 1 green apple, peeled
and chopped • 1 teaspoon fresh mint, chopped
• 1 teaspoon grated ginger • 1 teaspoon honey

• 1 glass of water • Ice
cubes (optional)

Method of preparation:

1. **Preparation of Ingredients:** • Peel and
cut the cucumber into slices. • Squeeze the juice from
the two lemons. • Chop the green apple. •
Finely chop the mint. • Grate
the ginger to get a teaspoon.

2. **Juice Assembly:**
• Place the cucumber slices, lemon juice, green apple, mint, ginger and honey in a blender.

3. **Adding Liquids:** • Pour
the glass of water over the ingredients in the blender.

4. **Beat Well:**
• Beat all ingredients until you obtain a smooth and homogeneous mixture.

5. **Adding Ice (Optional):** • If you
prefer, add ice cubes for a more refreshing experience.

6. **Serve Immediately:**
• Pour the cucumber and lemon detox juice into a glass and serve immediately.

Tip: Garnish the glass with a thin slice of cucumber or a mint leaf for a visually appealing touch. This detox
juice is excellent for hydration and contributes to the detoxification of the body.

Acerola Energy Juice

Ingredients:

• 1 cup of acerolas, seedless • 1 orange, peeled
and divided into segments • 1 apple, peeled and chopped
• 1 teaspoon of honey • 1 teaspoon of
chia (optional) • 1 glass of water
• Cubes of ice (optional)

Method of preparation:

1. **Preparation of Ingredients:** • Remove
   the seeds from the acerolas.
   • Peel the orange and separate it into segments. • Chop
   the apple.
2. **Juice Assembly:**
   • Place the acerolas, orange segments, apple, honey and chia (if using) in the
   blender.
3. **Adding Liquids:** • Pour
   the glass of water over the ingredients in the blender.
4. **Beat Well:**
   • Beat all ingredients until you obtain a smooth and homogeneous mixture.
5. **Adding Ice (Optional):** • If you
   prefer, add ice cubes for a more refreshing experience.
6. **Serve Immediately:**
   • Pour the acerola energy juice into a glass and serve immediately.

Tip: Decorate the glass with a few whole acerolas or a thin slice of orange for a visually appealing touch.
This energy juice is rich in vitamin C and nutrients that help boost energy naturally.

Professional Detox Green Salad

Ingredients:

• Lettuce

• Spinach •

Cucumber •

Celery •

Parsley •

Lemon and olive oil dressing

Step by step:

Step 1 - Preparation of the Vegetables:

• Carefully wash the lettuce and spinach under running water. • Tear lettuce and
spinach leaves into smaller pieces to make them easier to eat. • Peel and cut the cucumber into thin slices. •
Cut the celery into small pieces. • Finely chop the parsley.

Step 2 - Assembling the Salad:

• In a large bowl, combine the lettuce, spinach, cucumber, celery and parsley. • Make sure the
ingredients are evenly distributed.

Step 3 - Preparation of the Sauce:

• In a small bowl, mix fresh lemon juice with olive oil. Use a ratio of 2 parts olive oil to 1 part lemon juice. • Add
a pinch of salt and pepper to taste. • Stir well to emulsify the ingredients.

Step 4 - Finalization:

• Pour the dressing over the prepared green salad. • Gently toss
the vegetables to ensure the sauce coats all ingredients evenly.

Step 5 - Presentation:

• Serve the Detox Green Salad on individual plates or as a side dish. • Garnish with some parsley or
celery leaves for a finishing touch.

Pro Tips:

- Use fresh, high-quality ingredients to ensure flavor and benefits nutritional.

- Try adding chia seeds or flaxseeds for an added boost of fiber and omega-3s.

- Serve the salad immediately after adding the dressing to maintain the crunchiness of the salad. vegetables.

This Detox Green Salad not only provides a burst of flavor, but is also rich in essential nutrients to revitalize your body. Enjoy this healthy and delicious recipe as part of your wellness regimen!

Pro Tips:

Professional Detox Colorful Salad

Ingredients:

• Cherry tomatoes •
Red and yellow peppers • Grated carrots •
Grated beets • Arugula
• Yogurt sauce with herbs

Step by step:

Step 1 - Preparation of the Vegetables:

• Wash the cherry tomatoes and cut them in half. • Cut the
red and yellow pepper into thin strips. • Grate the carrot and beetroot,
ensuring a fine texture. • Carefully wash and dry the arugula.

Step 2 - Assembling the Salad:

• In a large bowl, combine the cherry tomatoes, bell pepper, grated carrot,
grated beetroot and arugula. •
Distribute the ingredients evenly in the bowl.

Step 3 - Preparation of the Yogurt Sauce with Herbs:

• In a small bowl, mix plain yogurt with chopped fresh herbs, such as
basil, parsley or mint. • Add a pinch
of salt and pepper to taste. • Stir well to ensure the herbs are
incorporated into the yogurt.

Step 4 - Finalization:

• Pour the yogurt sauce over the prepared colorful salad. • Gently toss the vegetables
to ensure the sauce coats all ingredients evenly.

Step 5 - Presentation:

• Serve the Colorful Detox Salad on individual plates or as a side dish. • Add a finishing touch with fresh
herb leaves or a pinch of pepper.

Pro Tips:

• Vary the colors of vegetables to ensure a variety of nutrients.

• Try adding sunflower or pumpkin seeds for a crunchy texture.

• Serve the salad on a large platter for a vibrant presentation at events
  specials.

This Colorful Detox Salad is not only visually stunning, but also offers a burst of fresh, healthy flavors. Enjoy this nutritious recipe as a delicious addition to your balanced lifestyle!

Professional Detox Quinoa Salad

Ingredients:

• Cooked quinoa •
Tomato
• Cucumber
• Coriander
• Avocado •
Lemon and olive oil dressing

Step by step:

Step 1 - Quinoa Preparation:

• Cook the quinoa according to the package instructions. • Let it cool before using
in salad.

Step 2 - Preparation of the Vegetables:

• Cut the tomatoes into medium cubes. • Peel and

cut the cucumber into thin slices. • Finely chop the coriander.
• Cut the avocado into cubes.

Step 3 - Assembling the Salad:

• In a large bowl, combine the cooked quinoa, tomatoes, cucumber, cilantro and
   avocado.
• Ensure that all ingredients are evenly distributed in the
   bowl.

Step 4 - Preparation of the Sauce:

• In a small bowl, mix fresh lemon juice with olive oil. Use a ratio of 2 parts olive oil to 1 part lemon juice. •
   Add a pinch of salt and pepper to taste. • Stir well to emulsify the ingredients.

Step 5 - Finalization:

• Pour the lemon dressing over the prepared quinoa salad. • Gently mix the
ingredients to ensure the sauce evenly coats the entire mixture.

Step 6 - Presentation:

• Serve the Detox Quinoa Salad on individual plates or as a side dish. • Garnish with coriander leaves for a fresh touch.

Pro Tips:

• Make sure to cook the quinoa until it is soft and loose. • Add a touch of cayenne pepper to the sauce for extra flavor. • This salad is an excellent option to prepare in advance and take with you.
healthy lunch box.

Enjoy this Detox Quinoa Salad, packed with proteins and nutrients, as a delicious and nutritious choice to promote your health and well-being.

Professional Detox Fruit Salad

Ingredients:

• Strawberries •
Pineapple •

Apple •
Grapes
• Mint •
Orange juice for drizzling

Step by step:

Step 1 - Fruit Preparation:

• Wash the strawberries and cut them into slices. •
Peel and cut the pineapple into small pieces. • Cut the apple into
cubes, removing the seeds.
• Wash the grapes and cut them in half.
• Finely chop the mint leaves.

Step 2 - Assembling the Salad:

• In a large bowl, combine the strawberries, pineapple, apple, grapes and mint. • Distribute the fruits
evenly in the bowl.

Step 3 - Preparation of the Orange Sauce:

• Squeeze fresh orange juice. • Water the fruits
with the orange juice, covering them completely.

Step 4 - Finalization:

• Gently stir the fruit to ensure the orange juice is well
distributed.

Step 5 - Presentation:

• Serve the Detox Fruit Salad in individual bowls. • Garnish with mint
leaves for a refreshing touch.

Pro Tips:

• Try adding a pinch of cinnamon or ginger to fruit to intensify the
flavors.

- Leave the salad in the fridge for a few minutes before serving for an experiment
  more refreshing.
- Vary fruits according to the season to ensure freshness and diversity.

This Detox Fruit Salad is a delicious and nutritious way to satisfy your sweet tooth while providing your body with essential vitamins and antioxidants.
Enjoy it as a light and revitalizing option for any occasion.

Professional Detox Lentil Salad

Ingredients:

• Cooked lentils
• Tomato •
Red onion • Cilantro

• Lemon •
Olive oil

Step by step:

Step 1 - Preparation of the Lentils:

• Cook the lentils according to the package instructions. • Let it cool before using in salad.

Step 2 - Preparation of the Vegetables:

• Cut the tomatoes into medium cubes. • Finely
chop the red onion. • Chop the coriander.

Step 3 - Assembling the Salad:

• In a large bowl, combine the cooked lentils, tomatoes, red onion and
    coriander.
• Ensure even distribution of ingredients in the bowl.

Step 4 - Preparation of the Lemon Sauce:

• Squeeze fresh lemon juice. • In a small
bowl, mix the lemon juice with olive oil. • Add a pinch of salt and pepper to taste. • Stir well
to emulsify the ingredients.

Step 5 - Finalization:

• Pour the lemon dressing over the prepared lentil salad. • Gently mix the ingredients
to ensure the sauce is combined.
    evenly distributed.

Step 6 - Presentation:

• Serve the Detox Lentil Salad on individual plates or as a side dish.

• Add a finishing touch with some coriander leaves for presentation.

Pro Tips:

• Make sure not to overcook the lentils to maintain a firm texture.
• Add minced garlic to the lemon sauce for extra flavor.
• This salad can be refrigerated for a few hours before serving to develop
  even more flavors.

Enjoy this Detox Lentil Salad as an option rich in protein and fiber, providing a healthy and satisfying meal for your body.

Professional Detox Cucumber Salad

Ingredients:

• Sliced cucumber • Tomato •
Red onion •
Basil • Apple cider
vinegar

Step by step:

Step 1 - Preparation of the Vegetables:

• Cut the cucumber into thin slices. • Cut the
tomatoes into medium cubes.
• Finely chop the red onion. • Chop the
basil.

Step 2 - Assembling the Salad:

• In a large bowl, combine the cucumber slices, tomatoes, red onion and
   basil.
• Make sure the ingredients are evenly distributed in the
   bowl.

Step 3 - Preparing the Apple Cider Vinegar Sauce:

• In a small bowl, mix the apple cider vinegar with a pinch of salt. • If desired, add a touch of honey
to balance the flavors. • Stir well to ensure a homogeneous mixture.

Step 4 - Finalization:

• Pour the apple cider vinegar dressing over the prepared cucumber salad. • Gently toss the
vegetables to ensure the sauce coats evenly.

Step 5 - Presentation:

• Serve the Detox Cucumber Salad on individual plates or as a side dish. • Garnish with basil leaves for a
fresh touch.

Pro Tips:

• Leave the salad in the fridge for a while before serving for a more flavorful experience.
   refreshing.

- Add freshly ground black pepper to the sauce for a touch of heat.
- This salad pairs well with grilled chicken breast for a heartier meal.
  substantial.

Enjoy this Detox Cucumber Salad as a light and hydrating option, perfect for revitalizing your body. Its refreshing combination of ingredients makes it a healthy and delicious choice.

Professional Detox Avocado Salad

Ingredients:

• Diced avocado

• Cherry tomatoes •
Arugula •
Chia seeds

• Lemon and olive oil dressing

Step by step:

Step 1 - Preparation of Ingredients:

• Cut the avocado into medium cubes. • Cut the
cherry tomatoes in half. • Carefully wash and
dry the arugula. • Prepare the chia seeds.

Step 2 - Assembling the Salad:

• In a large bowl, combine the diced avocado, cherry tomatoes, arugula and
Chia seeds.

• Make sure the ingredients are evenly distributed.

Step 3 - Preparation of the Lemon Sauce:

• Squeeze fresh lemon juice. • In a small
bowl, mix the lemon juice with olive oil. • Add a pinch of salt and pepper to taste. • Stir well
to emulsify the ingredients.

Step 4 - Finalization:

• Pour the lemon dressing over the prepared avocado salad. • Gently mix the
ingredients to ensure the sauce coats evenly
the whole salad.

Step 5 - Presentation:

• Serve the Detox Avocado Salad on individual plates or as a side dish. • Add a finishing touch with some chia
seeds on top.

Pro Tips:

- Make sure the avocado is ripe but firm to maintain its texture in the salad.

- Add a touch of honey to the lemon sauce for a sweet and sour flavor.

- This salad is an excellent source of healthy fats and essential nutrients.

Enjoy this Detox Avocado Salad as a delicious and nutritious option to promote your body's health. Its combination of fresh and tasty ingredients makes it a perfect choice for a balanced diet.

Professional Detox Kale Salad

Ingredients:

• Finely chopped cabbage • Grated
carrot • Sliced almonds
• Sesame seeds • Ginger
sauce

Step by step:

Step 1 - Preparation of Ingredients:

• Finely chop the cabbage, ensuring a fine texture. • Grate the carrot to a
delicate consistency. • Slice the almonds to add crunch. • Lightly
toast the sesame seeds in a frying pan, if desired.

Step 2 - Assembling the Salad:

• In a large bowl, combine the chopped kale, grated carrot, sliced almonds and
   Sesame.
• Make sure all ingredients are evenly distributed.

Step 3 - Preparation of the Ginger Sauce:

• Prepare ginger sauce by mixing grated fresh ginger with soy sauce. • Add a dash of honey for a bittersweet
touch. • Stir well to ensure a homogeneous combination.

Step 4 - Finalization:

• Pour the ginger dressing over the prepared kale salad. • Gently mix the ingredients to
ensure the sauce is evenly
   distributed.

Step 5 - Presentation:

• Serve the Detox Kale Salad on individual plates or as a side dish. • Decorate with some sliced almonds
on top.

Pro Tips:

• Massage the cabbage with a little olive oil before assembling the salad to soften it
   its fibers.

- Add a pinch of cayenne pepper to the ginger sauce for a kick
  spicy.
- This salad is an excellent option to accompany fish or chicken dishes
  grilled.

Enjoy this Detox Kale Salad as a healthy, nutrient-packed choice. Its vibrant flavor and mix of textures make it a delicious addition to your repertoire of detox recipes.

Professional Detox Pear Salad

Ingredients:

• Sliced pear
• Spinach • Nuts
• Feta cheese
• Honey and lemon
sauce

Step by step:

Step 1 - Preparation of Ingredients:

• Slice the pears into thin slices. •
Carefully wash and dry the spinach leaves. • Break or chop the nuts to
get smaller pieces. • Tear the feta cheese into small pieces.

Step 2 - Assembling the Salad:

• In a large bowl, combine the pear slices, spinach leaves, nuts and cheese
   feta.
• Ensure that all ingredients are evenly distributed in the bowl.

Step 3 - Preparation of the Honey and Lemon Sauce:

• In a small bowl, mix fresh honey with lemon juice. • Add a pinch of salt and pepper
to taste. • Stir well to create a homogeneous mixture.

Step 4 - Finalization:

• Pour the honey and lemon dressing over the prepared pear salad. • Gently mix the
ingredients to ensure the sauce is evenly
   distributed.

Step 5 - Presentation:

• Serve the Detox Pear Salad on individual plates or as a side dish. • Decorate with some whole walnuts
on top.

Pro Tips:

• Use ripe pears, but still firm, for a more pleasant texture. • Try adding chopped mint leaves to
the sauce for a touch of freshness.

• This salad pairs wonderfully with grilled chicken breast for a
more substantial meal.

Enjoy this Detox Pear Salad as an elegant and healthy option. Its combination
of sweet and savory flavors, together with the crunch of nuts, creates a delicious and
balanced gastronomic experience.

• This salad pairs wonderfully with grilled chicken breast for a
more substantial meal.

Professional Detox Broccoli Salad

Ingredients:

• Cooked broccoli
• Tomato •
Almonds • Raisins
• Yogurt sauce with
mustard

Step by step:

Step 1 - Preparation of Ingredients:

• Cook the broccoli until it is al dente. Cut them into small bouquets. • Cut the tomatoes into medium cubes.

• Slice the almonds to add crunch. • Make sure the raisins
are ready to use.

Step 2 - Assembling the Salad:

• In a large bowl, combine the cooked broccoli, tomatoes, almonds and grapes
   raisins.
• Ensure that all ingredients are evenly distributed in the
   bowl.

Step 3 - Preparation of the Yogurt Sauce with Mustard:

• In a small bowl, mix natural yogurt with mustard. • Add a pinch of salt and pepper
to taste. • Stir well to ensure a homogeneous mixture.

Step 4 - Finalization:

• Pour the yogurt-mustard dressing over the prepared broccoli salad. • Gently mix the ingredients to
ensure the sauce is evenly
   distributed.

Step 5 - Presentation:

• Serve the Detox Broccoli Salad on individual plates or as a side dish. • Decorate with some whole almonds
on top.

Pro Tips:

• Keep broccoli al dente to preserve its nutrients.

• Add a teaspoon of honey to the sauce for a touch of sweetness.
• This salad is an excellent option to prepare in advance and serve cold.

Enjoy this Detox Broccoli Salad as a nutritious and flavor-packed option.
Its combination of crunchy broccoli, almonds, and yogurt-mustard sauce creates a
healthy and satisfying taste experience.

Professional Detox Watermelon Salad

Ingredients:

• Cubed watermelon
• Goat cheese • Basil •
Olive oil

Step by step:

Step 1 - Preparation of Ingredients:

• Cut the watermelon into medium cubes.
• Break the goat cheese into small pieces. • Wash and dry the basil
leaves.

Step 2 - Assembling the Salad:

• In a large bowl, combine the watermelon cubes, goat cheese pieces and
    basil leaves.
• Make sure all ingredients are evenly distributed in the
    bowl.

Step 3 - Preparation of the Sauce:

• In a small bowl, mix olive oil with a pinch of salt. • Add a pinch of freshly ground black
pepper for a touch of heat. • Stir well to emulsify the ingredients.

Step 4 - Finalization:

• Drizzle the olive oil dressing over the prepared watermelon salad. • Gently mix
the ingredients to ensure the sauce is combined.
    evenly distributed.

Step 5 - Presentation:

• Serve the Detox Watermelon Salad on individual plates or as a side dish. • Garnish with additional basil
leaves for a finishing touch.

Pro Tips:

• Chill the watermelon cubes before assembling the salad for a refreshing touch. • Add a touch of balsamic
vinegar to the olive oil dressing for complexity
    of flavor.

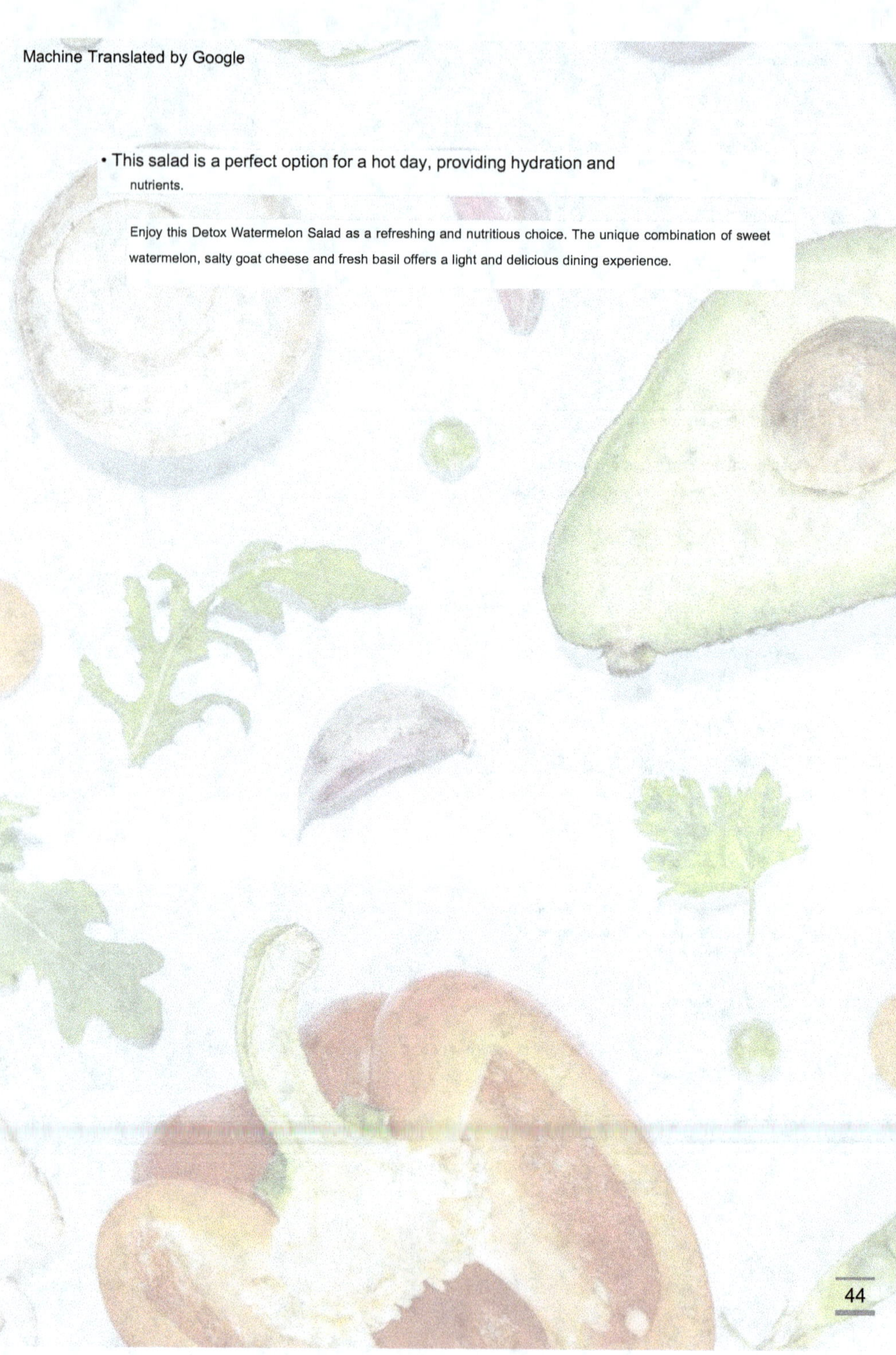

- This salad is a perfect option for a hot day, providing hydration and nutrients.

Enjoy this Detox Watermelon Salad as a refreshing and nutritious choice. The unique combination of sweet watermelon, salty goat cheese and fresh basil offers a light and delicious dining experience.

Professional Detox Seaweed Salad

Ingredients:

• Nori seaweed
• Cucumber
• Avocado •
Sesame • Soy
sauce

Step by step:

Step 1 - Preparation of Ingredients:

• Cut the nori seaweed into thin strips. •
Peel and cut the cucumber into thin slices. • Cut the avocado
into medium cubes. • Toast the sesame seeds
in a frying pan, if desired.

Step 2 - Assembling the Salad:

• In a large bowl, combine the nori seaweed strips, cucumber slices,
    avocado and sesame.
• Make sure all ingredients are evenly distributed in the
    bowl.

Step 3 - Preparation of the Soy Sauce:

• In a small bowl, mix soy sauce with a pinch of fresh ginger
    grated.
• Add a dash of sesame oil for additional flavor. • Stir well to create a homogeneous
mixture.

Step 4 - Finalization:

• Pour soy sauce over the prepared seaweed salad. • Gently mix the ingredients
to ensure the sauce is evenly
    distributed.

Step 5 - Presentation:

• Serve the Detox Seaweed Salad on individual plates or as a side dish. • Decorate with an additional
touch of sesame seeds on top.

Pro Tips:

• Use fresh or rehydrated seaweed, depending on availability.
• Add some wasabi to the soy sauce for a spicy kick.
• This salad is an excellent source of minerals and antioxidants.

Enjoy this Detox Seaweed Salad as a unique option full of health benefits. Its distinct flavor profile and rich nutrient content make it a delicious and nutritious choice for a balanced diet.

Professional Detox Bean Salad

Ingredients:

• Cooked black beans •
Cooked corn • Red
bell pepper • Cilantro

• Avocado •
Lemon and olive oil dressing

Step by step:

Step 1 - Preparation of Ingredients:

• Cook black beans until tender, following package instructions. • Cook the corn until it is cooked. • Cut
the red pepper into medium cubes. • Finely chop the
coriander. • Cut the avocado into medium cubes.

Step 2 - Assembling the Salad:

• In a large bowl, combine cooked black beans, cooked corn, bell peppers
red, coriander and avocado cubes. • Ensure that
all ingredients are evenly distributed in the
bowl.

Step 3 - Preparation of the Sauce:

• In a small bowl, mix fresh lemon juice with olive oil. Use a ratio of 2 parts olive oil to 1 part lemon juice. •
Add a pinch of salt and pepper to taste. • Stir well to emulsify the ingredients.

Step 4 - Finalization:

• Pour the lemon dressing over the prepared bean salad. • Gently mix the
ingredients to ensure the sauce is evenly
distributed.

Step 5 - Presentation:

• Serve the Detox Bean Salad on individual plates or as a side dish. • Add some additional coriander leaves
on top for garnish.

Pro Tips:

• Try adding a pinch of cumin to the sauce for a kick of flavor
extra.

• This salad is an option rich in protein and fiber, perfect as a main dish or side dish.

• Prepare the salad in advance to allow the flavors to develop.

Enjoy this Detox Bean Salad as a substantial and healthy option. With a delicious mix of ingredients, it provides a nutritious meal that is both satisfying and full of health benefits.

Professional Detox Zucchini Salad

Ingredients:

• Zucchini into thin strips
• Cherry tomatoes •
Ricotta cheese •
Basil • Sliced
almonds • Lemon vinaigrette

Step by step:

Step 1 - Preparation of Ingredients:

• Use a vegetable peeler to create thin strips of zucchini. • Cut the cherry tomatoes in half. •
Crumble the ricotta cheese into small pieces.
• Finely chop the basil leaves. • Toast the sliced almonds in a
frying pan, if desired.

Step 2 - Assembling the Salad:

• In a large bowl, combine the zucchini strips, cherry tomatoes, ricotta cheese, basil and sliced almonds. •
Ensure that all ingredients are evenly
distributed in the bowl.

Step 3 - Preparation of the Lemon Vinaigrette:

• In a small bowl, mix fresh lemon juice with olive oil. • Add a pinch of salt and pepper to taste. •
Stir well to emulsify the ingredients.

Step 4 - Finalization:

• Drizzle the lemon vinaigrette over the prepared zucchini salad. • Gently mix the
ingredients to ensure the vinaigrette is
evenly distributed.

Step 5 - Presentation:

• Serve the Detox Zucchini Salad on individual plates or as a side dish. • Decorate with additional basil leaves
and sliced almonds on top.

Pro Tips:

- Season the zucchini with salt and let it rest for a few minutes to remove the excess moisture before assembling the salad.
- Add lemon zest to the vinaigrette to intensify the citrus flavor.
- This salad is a light and tasty choice, perfect for hotter days.

Enjoy this Detox Zucchini Salad as a fresh and nutritious option. With a mix of textures and flavors, it offers a delicious gastronomic experience while promoting health and well-being.

Professional Detox Strawberry Salad

Ingredients:

• Sliced strawberries •
Spinach • Goat
cheese • Sliced almonds
• Honey and balsamic
vinaigrette

Step by step:

Step 1 - Preparation of Ingredients:

• Slice the strawberries into thin slices. • Carefully
wash and dry the spinach leaves. • Break the goat cheese into small
pieces. • Lightly toast the sliced almonds in a frying pan, if desired.

Step 2 - Assembling the Salad:

• In a large bowl, combine the strawberry slices, spinach leaves, cheese and
goat and sliced almonds.
• Make sure all ingredients are evenly distributed in the
bowl.

Step 3 - Preparation of the Balsamic and Honey Vinaigrette:

• In a small bowl, mix balsamic vinegar with honey. • Add a pinch of salt and
pepper to taste. • Stir well to create a homogeneous mixture.

Step 4 - Finalization:

• Drizzle the honey-balsamic vinaigrette over the prepared strawberry salad. • Gently mix the
ingredients to ensure the vinaigrette is smooth.
evenly distributed.

Step 5 - Presentation:

• Serve the Detox Strawberry Salad on individual plates or as a side dish. • Garnish with some spinach leaves
and additional strawberries on top.

Pro Tips:

• Add a touch of fresh mint to the vinaigrette for a refreshing taste.

• Try substituting feta cheese for goat cheese for a variation in flavor.
• This salad is a vibrant and delicious choice for a light meal.

Enjoy this Detox Strawberry Salad as a sweet and healthy option. With fresh ingredients and a balanced mix of flavors, it offers a nutritious and delicious culinary experience.

Professional Detox Pumpkin Salad

Ingredients:

• Pumpkin cut into cubes

• Cooked quinoa •

Spinach •
Roasted pumpkin seeds

• Mustard and honey sauce

Step by step:

Step 1 - Preparation of Ingredients:

• Cut the pumpkin into cubes and cook until it is soft. • Cook the quinoa
according to the package instructions. • Carefully wash and dry the spinach leaves.

• Toast the pumpkin seeds in a skillet, if desired.

Step 2 - Assembling the Salad:

• In a large bowl, combine the pumpkin cubes, cooked quinoa,
   spinach and roasted pumpkin seeds.

• Ensure that all ingredients are evenly distributed in the
   bowl.

Step 3 - Preparation of the Mustard and Honey Sauce:

• In a small bowl, mix mustard, honey and olive oil. • Add a pinch of salt and pepper
to taste. • Stir well to create a homogeneous mixture.

Step 4 - Finalization:

• Drizzle the honey mustard dressing over the prepared pumpkin salad. • Gently mix the
ingredients to ensure the sauce is combined.
   evenly distributed.

Step 5 - Presentation:

• Serve the Detox Pumpkin Salad on individual plates or as a side dish. • Garnish with some extra spinach
leaves and pumpkin seeds on top.

Pro Tips:

• Use different varieties of pumpkin for a combination of colors and flavors.

• Add a splash of balsamic vinegar to the dressing for added complexity. • This salad is an excellent source of fiber and essential nutrients.

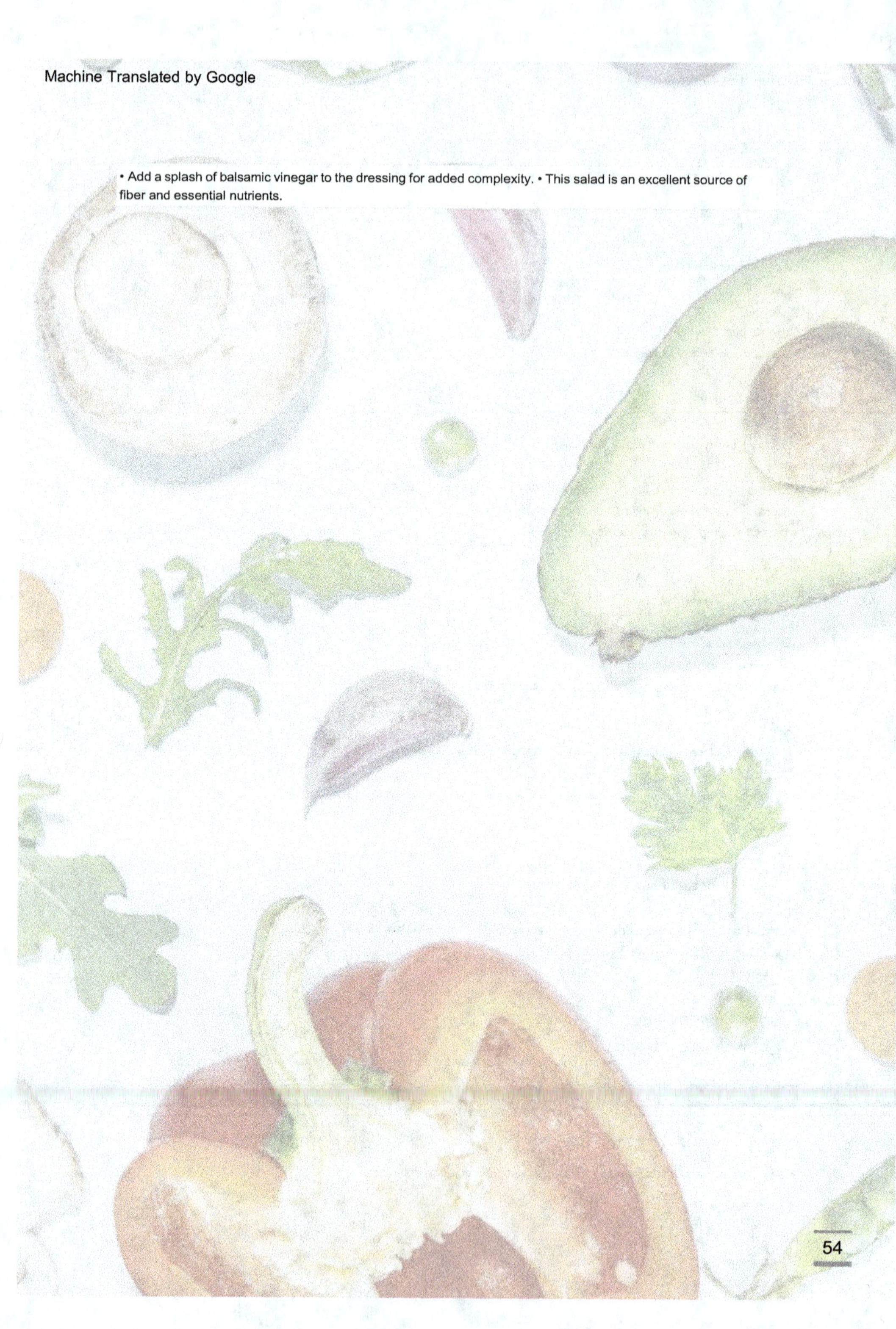

Professional Detox Mushroom Salad

Ingredients:

• Assorted mushrooms (shiitake, white mushrooms, etc.), sliced • Baby spinach •
Cherry tomatoes •
Feta cheese •
Chopped nuts •
Lemon vinaigrette
dressing

Step by step:

Step 1 - Preparation of Ingredients:

• Slice the mushrooms into thin pieces. • Carefully
wash and dry the baby spinach leaves. • Cut the cherry tomatoes in half. •
Tear the feta cheese into small pieces. •
Chop the nuts.

Step 2 - Assembling the Salad:

• In a large bowl, combine the sliced mushrooms, baby spinach, cherry tomatoes,
feta cheese and chopped walnuts.
• Make sure all ingredients are evenly distributed in the
bowl.

Step 3 - Preparation of the Lemon Vinaigrette Dressing:

• In a small bowl, mix fresh lemon juice with olive oil. • Add a pinch of salt and pepper to taste.
• Stir well to emulsify the ingredients.

Step 4 - Finalization:

• Drizzle the lemon vinaigrette dressing over the prepared mushroom salad. • Gently mix the
ingredients to ensure the vinaigrette is smooth.
evenly distributed.

Step 5 - Presentation:

• Serve the Detox Mushroom Salad on individual plates or as a side dish. • Garnish with some additional
spinach leaves and walnuts on top.

Pro Tips:

• Experiment with different types of mushrooms for a variety of flavors and textures. • Add a touch of honey to vinaigrette dressing for a sweet and sour flavor. • This salad is an option rich in proteins and nutrients, perfect for a meal healthy.

Professional Detox Asparagus Salad

Ingredients:

• Fresh asparagus • Grape
tomatoes • Boiled
eggs • Sliced almonds

• Dijon mustard sauce

Step by step:

Step 1 - Preparation of Ingredients:

• Cut the tough stalks from the asparagus and cook in boiling water until al dente. In
 Then immerse them in ice water to stop the cooking.
• Cut the grape tomatoes in half. • Cook and
chop the eggs.

Step 2 - Assembling the Salad:

• In a large bowl, combine the cooked asparagus, grape tomatoes and hard-boiled eggs. • Make sure all
ingredients are evenly distributed in the
 bowl.

Step 3 - Preparing the Dijon Mustard Sauce:

• In a small bowl, mix Dijon mustard with olive oil. • Add a pinch of salt and pepper to taste. •
Stir well to emulsify the ingredients.

Step 4 - Finalization:

• Drizzle Dijon mustard dressing over the prepared asparagus salad. • Gently mix the ingredients
to ensure the sauce is combined.
 evenly distributed.

Step 5 - Presentation:

• Serve the Detox Asparagus Salad on individual plates or as a side dish. • Sprinkle sliced almonds on top to
add a crunchy touch.

Pro Tips:

• Cook asparagus just until al dente to maintain vibrant texture and color. • Add a splash of white wine vinegar to
the sauce for extra flavor.

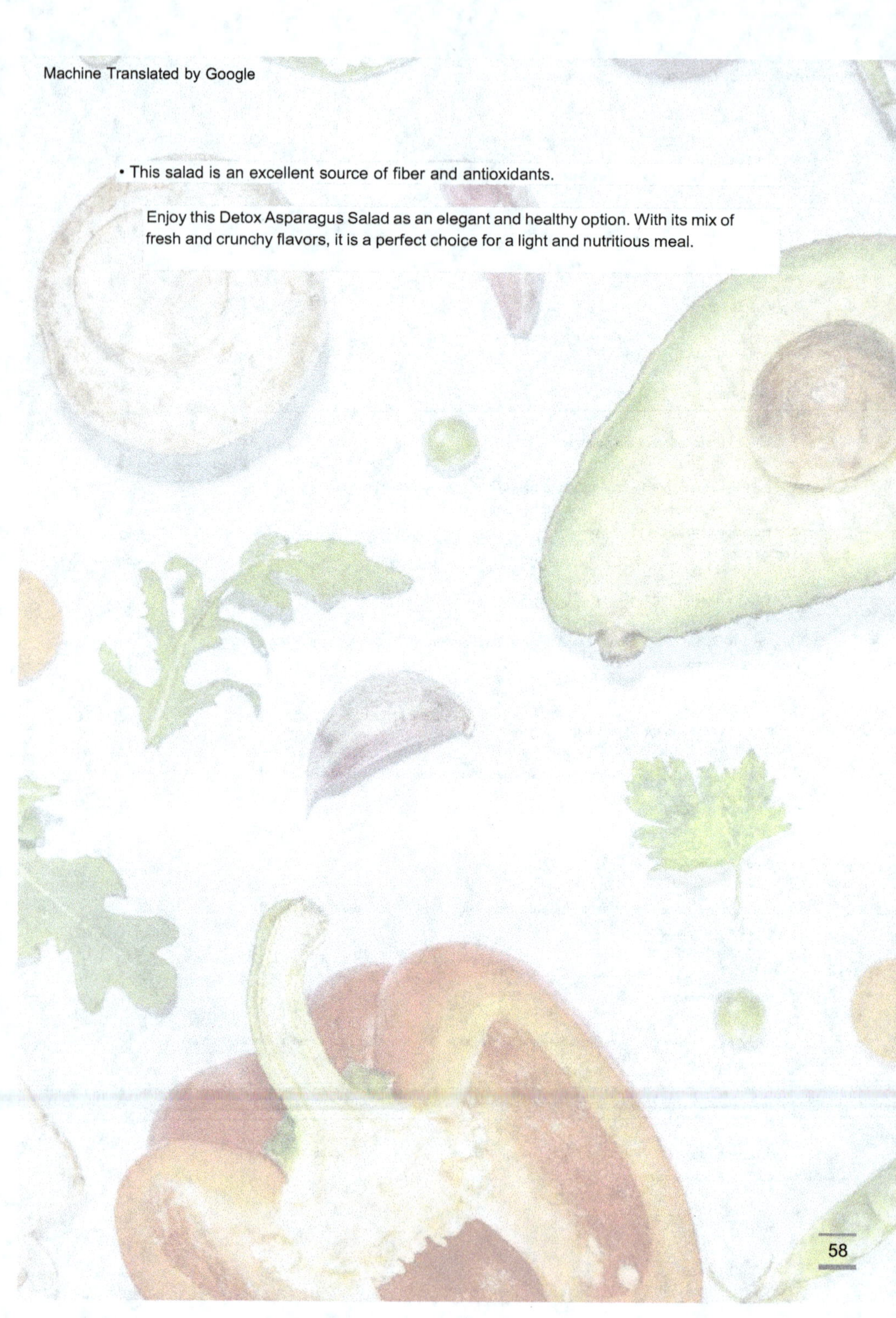

• This salad is an excellent source of fiber and antioxidants.

Enjoy this Detox Asparagus Salad as an elegant and healthy option. With its mix of fresh and crunchy flavors, it is a perfect choice for a light and nutritious meal.

Detox Green Broth with Kale and Butter

Ingredients:

• 2 cups of chopped kale • 1 medium onion,
chopped • 2 cloves of garlic,
chopped • 1 medium sweet potato,
diced
• 1 carrot, sliced • 1 stalk of
celery, chopped • Salt and
pepper to taste • 1 liter of
vegetable broth

Method of preparation:

Step 1: Preparation of Ingredients

• Wash and chop the kale. • Chop the onion
and garlic cloves. • Peel and cut the sweet potato
into cubes. • Cut the carrot into slices. • Chop the celery
stalk.

Step 2: Sautéing the Aromatics

• In a large pan, heat a tablespoon of olive oil over medium heat. • Saute the onion and garlic until
golden and aromatic.

Step 3: Adding Vegetables

• Add the carrot slices, sweet potato cubes and celery stalk to the pan.
Saute for a few minutes.

Step 4: Incorporating the Kale

• Add 2 cups of chopped kale. Stir until the cabbage starts to wilt.

Step 5: Seasoning

• Season with salt and pepper to taste. Adjust as needed.

Step 6: Adding Broth

• Pour the liter of vegetable broth into the pan. Stir well to incorporate the
Ingredients.

Step 7: Cooking

• Let the mixture boil. Reduce heat and simmer for 15-20 minutes, until vegetables become soft.

Step 8: Adjusting the Flavor

• Taste and adjust seasoning if necessary.

Step 9: Liquidification

• Use an immersion blender to obtain a smooth, velvety green broth.

Step 10: Serving

• Serve the Caldo Verde Detox with a drizzle of olive oil and some kale leaves as decoration.

Step 11: Enjoy your nutritious detox soup!

Pro Tip: Serve with a slice of whole grain bread for a complete meal and

Carrot and Celery Soup

Ingredients:

• 3 medium carrots, peeled and sliced • 2 stalks of celery,
chopped • 1 medium onion,
chopped • 2 cloves of garlic,
chopped • 1 diced potato • 1 liter of
vegetable broth • Salt and
pepper to taste

Method of preparation:

Step 1: Preparation of Ingredients

• Peel and slice the carrots. • Chop the
celery stalks. • Chop the onion
and garlic cloves. • Cut the potato into cubes.

Step 2: Sautéing Aromatics

• In a large pan, heat a tablespoon of olive oil over medium heat. • Saute the onion and garlic until
golden and aromatic.

Step 3: Adding Vegetables

• Add the carrots, celery stalks and potatoes to the pan. Saute for a few minutes.

Step 4: Incorporating Broth

• Pour the liter of vegetable broth into the pan. Stir well to incorporate the
Ingredients.

Step 5: Seasoning

• Season with salt and pepper to taste. Adjust as needed.

Step 6: Cooking

• Let the mixture boil. Reduce heat and simmer for 15-20 minutes, until vegetables
become soft.

Step 7: Adjusting the Flavor

- Taste and adjust seasoning if necessary.

Step 8: Liquidification

- Use an immersion blender to obtain a creamy, homogeneous soup.

Step 9: Serving

- Serve the Carrot and Celery Soup in individual bowls.

Step 10: Optional Decoration

- Add a pinch of pepper or celery leaves to decorate.

Step 11: Enjoy this comforting and nutritious soup!

Pro Tip: Try serving with a touch of plain yogurt or croutons for extra texture.

Creamed Spinach with Leek

Ingredients:

• 200g fresh spinach • 1 medium
leek, sliced • 1 diced potato • 2 cloves
of garlic, chopped • 1 liter
of vegetable broth • Salt and pepper
to taste

Method of preparation:

Step 1: Preparation of Ingredients

• Wash and chop the spinach. •
Slice the leek. • Cut the
potato into cubes. • Chop the garlic
cloves.

Step 2: Sautéing Aromatics

• Heat a tablespoon of olive oil in a large pan over medium heat. • Saute the leeks and garlic until
golden and aromatic.

Step 3: Adding Vegetables

• Add the spinach and potatoes to the pan. Saute for a few minutes.

Step 4: Incorporating Broth

• Pour the liter of vegetable broth into the pan. Stir to incorporate the ingredients.

Step 5: Seasoning

• Season with salt and pepper to taste. Adjust as needed.

Step 6: Cooking

• Let the mixture boil. Reduce heat and simmer for 15-20 minutes, until vegetables
become soft.

Step 7: Adjusting the Flavor

• Taste and adjust seasoning if necessary.

Step 8: Liquidification

• Use an immersion blender to obtain a smooth, homogeneous cream.

Step 9: Serving

• Serve the Creamed Spinach and Leeks in individual bowls.

Step 10: Optional Decoration

• Add a pinch of black pepper or a drizzle of olive oil for a final touch.

Step 11: Indulge in this nourishing and comforting cream!

Pro Tip: Serve with croutons or a sprinkle of nutmeg to enhance the flavors.

Lentil Soup with Vegetables

Ingredients:

• 1 cup of lentils
• 1 chopped carrot • 1
chopped onion • 2
chopped garlic cloves • 1 chopped
zucchini • 1 liter of vegetable
broth • Seasonings to taste

Method of preparation:

Step 1: Preparation of Ingredients

• Wash the lentils. • Chop
the carrot, onion, garlic cloves and zucchini.

Step 2: Sautéing Aromatics

• In a large pan, heat a tablespoon of olive oil over medium heat. • Sauté the onion and garlic until
golden and aromatic.

Step 3: Adding Vegetables and Lentils

• Add the carrot, zucchini and lentils to the pan. Saute for a few minutes.

Step 4: Incorporating Broth

• Pour the liter of vegetable broth into the pan. Stir to incorporate the ingredients.

Step 5: Seasoning

• Add seasonings to taste. It may include pepper, cumin or fresh herbs.

Step 6: Cooking

• Let the mixture boil. Reduce heat and simmer for 25-30 minutes, until lentils and
the vegetables become soft.

Step 7: Adjusting the Flavor

• Taste and adjust seasoning if necessary.

Step 8: Serving

• Serve Lentil Soup with Vegetables in individual bowls.

Step 9: Optional Decoration

• Add fresh parsley leaves or chives for a touch of freshness.

Step 10: Enjoy this nutritious and flavor-packed soup!

Pro Tip: Serve with a slice of whole grain bread or croutons for a more substantial experience.

Roasted Tomato Soup with Basil

Ingredients:

• 6 ripe tomatoes
• 1 chopped onion • 3
chopped garlic cloves • Fresh basil
leaves • 1 liter of vegetable broth • Salt
and pepper to taste

Method of preparation:

Step 1: Preparation of Ingredients

• Wash and cut the tomatoes in half.
• Chop the onion and garlic cloves. • Reserve
some basil leaves for decoration.

Step 2: Roasting the Tomatoes

• Preheat the oven to 200°C. • Place the
tomatoes on a baking tray, drizzle with olive oil and roast for 25-30 minutes, until they are soft and lightly golden.

Step 3: Sautéing Aromatics

• In a pan, heat a tablespoon of olive oil over medium heat. • Saute the onion and garlic until
golden and aromatic.

Step 4: Adding Roasted Tomatoes

• Add the roasted tomatoes to the pan. Shake well.

Step 5: Incorporating Broth

• Pour the liter of vegetable broth into the pan. Stir to incorporate the ingredients.

Step 6: Seasoning

• Season with salt and pepper to taste. Add some basil leaves.

Step 7: Cooking

• Let the mixture boil. Reduce heat and simmer for 15-20 minutes to bring out the flavors.
   flavors.

Step 8: Adjusting the Flavor

• Taste and adjust seasoning if necessary.

Step 9: Liquidification

• Use an immersion blender to obtain a smoother consistency.

Step 10: Serving

• Serve the Roasted Tomato and Basil Soup in individual bowls.

Step 11: Optional Decoration

• Add fresh basil leaves over the soup before serving.

Step 12: Enjoy this soup rich in flavors!

Pro Tip: Serve with croutons or a sprinkle of Parmesan cheese for an extra kick.

Cauliflower Cream with Turmeric

Ingredients:

• 1 medium cauliflower

• 1 chopped onion • 2
chopped garlic cloves • 1 teaspoon
of turmeric

• 1 liter of vegetable broth • Salt and
pepper to taste

Method of preparation:

Step 1: Preparation of Ingredients

• Separate the cauliflower florets. • Chop the
onion and garlic cloves.

Step 2: Sautéing Aromatics

• In a large pan, heat a tablespoon of olive oil over medium heat. • Saute the onion and garlic until
golden and aromatic.

Step 3: Adding Cauliflower

• Add the cauliflower florets to the pan. Saute for a few minutes.

Step 4: Incorporating Turmeric

• Add turmeric to the mixture. Stir well to distribute evenly.

Step 5: Adding Broth

• Pour the liter of vegetable broth into the pan. Stir to incorporate the ingredients.

Step 6: Seasoning

• Season with salt and pepper to taste. Adjust as needed.

Step 7: Cooking

• Let the mixture boil. Reduce heat and simmer for 15-20 minutes, until cauliflower
become soft.

Step 8: Adjusting the Flavor

• Taste and adjust seasoning if necessary.

Step 9: Liquidification

• Use an immersion blender to obtain a smooth cream.

Step 10: Serving

• Serve the Cauliflower Cream with Turmeric in individual bowls.

Step 11: Optional Decoration

• Add a touch of olive oil or sprinkle some turmeric before serving.

Step 12: Enjoy this creamy, comforting soup!

Pro Tip: Serve with croutons or a drizzle of cream for added texture.
extra.

Beetroot Soup with Mint

Ingredients:

• 2 medium beets, peeled and chopped • 1 onion, chopped
• 2 cloves of garlic,
chopped • Fresh mint leaves

• 1 liter of vegetable broth • Salt and
pepper to taste

Method of preparation:

Step 1: Preparation of Ingredients

• Peel and chop the beets. • Chop the onion
and garlic cloves. • Reserve some mint leaves
for decoration.

Step 2: Sautéing Aromatics

• In a large pan, heat a tablespoon of olive oil over medium heat. • Saute the onion and garlic until
golden and aromatic.

Step 3: Adding Beets

• Add the beets to the pan. Saute for a few minutes.

Step 4: Incorporating Broth

• Pour the liter of vegetable broth into the pan. Stir to incorporate the ingredients.

Step 5: Seasoning

• Season with salt and pepper to taste. Add some mint leaves.

Step 6: Cooking

• Let the mixture boil. Reduce heat and simmer for 20-25 minutes, until beets
become soft.

Step 7: Adjusting the Flavor

• Taste and adjust seasoning if necessary.

Step 8: Liquidification

• Use an immersion blender to obtain a smooth consistency.

Step 9: Serving

• Serve the Beetroot Soup with Mint in individual bowls.

Step 10: Optional Decoration

• Add fresh mint leaves over the soup before serving.

Step 11: Enjoy this vibrant and nutritious soup!

Pro Tip: Top with a spoonful of Greek yogurt for an added creamy texture.

Chickpea Soup with Spinach

Ingredients:

• 1 cup of cooked chickpeas • 2 cups of
spinach leaves • 1 chopped onion • 2
chopped garlic cloves •
1 diced carrot • 1 liter of vegetable
broth • Salt and pepper to taste

Method of preparation:

Step 1: Preparation of Ingredients

• Pre-cook the chickpeas until soft. • Wash the spinach leaves. • Chop
the onion, garlic cloves and carrot.

Step 2: Sautéing Aromatics

• Heat a tablespoon of olive oil in a large pan over medium heat. • Saute the onion and garlic until
golden and aromatic.

Step 3: Adding Vegetables and Chickpeas

• Add the carrot, cooked chickpeas and spinach leaves to the pan. Saute for a few minutes.

Step 4: Incorporating Broth

• Pour the liter of vegetable broth into the pan. Stir to incorporate the ingredients.

Step 5: Seasoning

• Season with salt and pepper to taste. Adjust as needed.

Step 6: Cooking

• Let the mixture boil. Reduce heat and simmer for 15-20 minutes, until vegetables
become soft.

Step 7: Adjusting the Flavor

• Taste and adjust seasoning if necessary.

Step 8: Blending (Optional)

• If you prefer, use an immersion blender to obtain a thicker consistency. creamy.

Step 9: Serving

• Serve the Chickpea and Spinach Soup in individual bowls.

Step 10: Optional Decoration

• Add a pinch of freshly ground black pepper or a drizzle of olive oil.

Step 11: Enjoy this nutritious and comforting soup!

Pro Tip: Try finishing with a squeeze of lemon juice to enhance the flavors.

Vegetable Broth with Quinoa

Ingredients:

• 1 cup of washed quinoa • 2 sliced
carrots • 2 chopped celery stalks

• 1 chopped onion • 2 chopped
garlic cloves • 1 liter of
vegetable broth • Salt and pepper
to taste

Method of preparation:

Step 1: Preparation of Ingredients

• Wash the quinoa well under running water. • Cut
the carrots into slices. • Chop the celery

stalks, onion and garlic cloves.

Step 2: Sautéing Aromatics

• Heat a tablespoon of olive oil in a large pan over medium heat. • Saute the onion and garlic until
golden and aromatic.

Step 3: Adding Vegetables and Quinoa

• Add the carrots, celery and quinoa to the pan. Saute for a few minutes.

Step 4: Incorporating Broth

• Pour the liter of vegetable broth into the pan. Stir to incorporate the ingredients.

Step 5: Seasoning

• Season with salt and pepper to taste. Adjust as needed.

Step 6: Cooking

• Let the mixture boil. Reduce heat and simmer for 15-20 minutes, until vegetables and
quinoa become soft.

Step 7: Adjusting the Flavor

• Taste and adjust seasoning if necessary.

Step 8: Serving

• Serve the Vegetable Broth with Quinoa in individual bowls.

Step 9: Optional Decoration

• Add fresh parsley leaves or chives for a touch of freshness.

Step 10: Enjoy this comforting, nutrient-packed broth!

Pro Tip: Try drizzling with extra virgin olive oil before serving.

Zucchini Soup with Cilantro

Ingredients:

• 3 medium zucchini, cut into cubes • 1 chopped onion •
2 chopped garlic cloves
• 1 diced potato

• 1 liter of vegetable broth • Fresh
coriander leaves
• Salt and pepper to taste

Method of preparation:

Step 1: Preparation of Ingredients

• Cut the zucchini into cubes. • Chop the
onion and garlic cloves. • Cut the potato into
cubes.
• Set aside some coriander leaves for decoration.

Step 2: Sautéing Aromatics

• Heat a tablespoon of olive oil in a large pan over medium heat. • Saute the onion and garlic until
golden and aromatic.

Step 3: Adding Vegetables

• Add the zucchini and potatoes to the pan. Saute for a few minutes.

Step 4: Incorporating Broth

• Pour the liter of vegetable broth into the pan. Stir to incorporate the ingredients.

Step 5: Seasoning

• Season with salt and pepper to taste. Adjust as needed.

Step 6: Cooking

• Let the mixture boil. Reduce heat and simmer for 15-20 minutes, until vegetables
become soft.

Step 7: Adjusting the Flavor

• Taste and adjust seasoning if necessary.

Step 8: Blending (Optional)

• Use an immersion blender to obtain a creamier consistency.

Step 9: Serving

• Serve Zucchini Soup with Cilantro in individual bowls.

Step 10: Optional Decoration

• Add fresh coriander leaves over the soup before serving.

Step 11: Enjoy this light and flavorful soup!

Pro Tip: Try drizzling with olive oil or adding a squeeze of lemon before serving.

Asparagus Cream with Lemon

Ingredients:

• 500g fresh asparagus, with ends trimmed • 1 chopped onion • 2 chopped
garlic cloves • 1 diced
potato

• 1 liter of vegetable broth • Juice and
zest of 1 lemon • Salt and pepper
to taste

Method of preparation:

Step 1: Preparation of Ingredients

• Cut the asparagus into small pieces. • Chop the onion
and garlic cloves. • Cut the potato into cubes.

• Grate the zest and squeeze the juice from the lemon.

Step 2: Sautéing Aromatics

• Heat a tablespoon of olive oil in a large pan over medium heat. • Saute the onion and garlic until
golden and aromatic.

Step 3: Adding Vegetables

• Add the asparagus and potatoes to the pan. Saute for a few minutes.

Step 4: Incorporating Broth

• Pour the liter of vegetable broth into the pan. Stir to incorporate the ingredients.

Step 5: Seasoning

• Season with salt and pepper to taste. Add the lemon juice.

Step 6: Cooking

• Let the mixture boil. Reduce heat and simmer for 15-20 minutes, until vegetables
become soft.

Step 7: Adjusting the Flavor

• Taste and adjust seasoning if necessary.

Step 8: Liquidification

• Use an immersion blender to obtain a smooth cream.

Step 9: Serving

• Serve the Asparagus Cream with Lemon in individual bowls.

Step 10: Optional Decoration

• Add a touch of lemon zest or a drizzle of olive oil.

Step 11: Indulge in this delicate and fresh cream!

Pro Tip: Try adding a handful of fresh basil leaves before serving for an extra kick of flavor.

Broccoli Soup with Saffron

Ingredients:

• 1 bunch of broccoli, separated into florets • 1 chopped
onion • 2 chopped garlic
cloves • 1 diced potato

• 1 liter of vegetable broth • 1 teaspoon
of turmeric • Salt and pepper to taste

Method of preparation:

Step 1: Preparation of Ingredients

• Separate the broccoli florets. • Chop the
onion and garlic cloves. • Cut the potato into
cubes.

Step 2: Sautéing Aromatics

• Heat a tablespoon of olive oil in a large pan over medium heat. • Saute the onion and garlic until
golden and aromatic.

Step 3: Adding Vegetables

• Add the broccoli florets and potatoes to the pan. Saute for a few minutes.

Step 4: Incorporating Broth

• Pour the liter of vegetable broth into the pan. Stir to incorporate the ingredients.

Step 5: Adding Turmeric

• Add saffron to the mixture. Stir well to distribute evenly.

Step 6: Seasoning

• Season with salt and pepper to taste. Adjust as needed.

Step 7: Cooking

• Let the mixture boil. Reduce heat and simmer for 15-20 minutes, until vegetables
become soft.

Step 8: Adjusting the Flavor

• Taste and adjust seasoning if necessary.

Step 9: Blending (Optional)

• If you prefer, use an immersion blender to obtain a thicker consistency.
creamy.

Step 10: Serving

• Serve the Saffron Broccoli Soup in individual bowls.

Step 11: Optional Decoration

• Add an extra pinch of saffron over the soup before serving.

Step 12: Enjoy this nutritious and colorful soup!

Pro Tip: Serve with croutons or a drizzle of olive oil for a finishing touch.

Leek Soup with Sweet Potatoes

Ingredients:

• 2 leeks, white and light green parts, sliced • 2 medium sweet
potatoes, peeled and cut into cubes • 1 chopped onion • 2 chopped garlic
cloves • 1 liter of
vegetable broth • 1 teaspoon of
olive oil olive

• Salt and pepper to taste

Method of preparation:

Step 1: Preparation of Ingredients

• Slice the leeks, cut the sweet potatoes into cubes, chop the onion and cloves
garlic.

Step 2: Sautéing Aromatics

• Heat the olive oil in a large pan over medium heat. • Saute the onion and garlic until
golden and aromatic.

Step 3: Adding Leeks and Sweet Potatoes

• Add the sliced leeks and sweet potatoes to the pan. Sauté for a few
minutes.

Step 4: Incorporating Broth

• Pour the liter of vegetable broth into the pan. Stir to incorporate the ingredients.

Step 5: Seasoning

• Season with salt and pepper to taste. Shake well.

Step 6: Cooking

• Let the mixture boil. Reduce the heat and simmer for 20-25 minutes, until the potatoes
sweets become soft.

Step 7: Adjusting the Flavor

• Taste and adjust seasoning if necessary.

Step 8: Blending (Optional)

• Use an immersion blender to obtain a creamier consistency if
to prefer.

Step 9: Serving

• Serve the Leek and Sweet Potato Soup in individual bowls.

Step 10: Optional Decoration

• Add a drizzle of olive oil or raw leek leaves for a visual touch.

Step 11: Enjoy this comforting, flavor-packed soup!

Pro Tip: Serve with toasted whole grain bread for a more substantial experience.

Mushroom Soup with Rosemary

Ingredients:

• 300g of assorted mushrooms, sliced • 1 chopped
onion • 2 chopped garlic
cloves • 1 diced potato

• 1 liter of vegetable broth • 1 sprig of
fresh rosemary

• 1 tablespoon olive oil • Salt and pepper to taste

Method of preparation:

Step 1: Preparation of Ingredients

• Slice the mushrooms, chop the onion, cut the potato into cubes and separate the rosemary.

Step 2: Sautéing Aromatics

• Heat the olive oil in a large pan over medium heat. • Saute the onion and garlic until
golden and aromatic.

Step 3: Adding Mushrooms and Potatoes

• Add the sliced mushrooms and potatoes to the pan. Saute for a few minutes.

Step 4: Incorporating Broth

• Pour the liter of vegetable broth into the pan. Stir to incorporate the ingredients.

Step 5: Seasoning

• Add the rosemary sprig, salt and pepper to taste. Shake well.

Step 6: Cooking

• Let the mixture boil. Reduce heat and simmer for 15-20 minutes, until potatoes
become soft.

Step 7: Adjusting the Flavor

• Taste and adjust seasoning if necessary.

Step 8: Removing the Rosemary

• Remove the rosemary sprig from the soup before proceeding.

Step 9: Serving

• Serve the Rosemary Mushroom Soup in individual bowls.

Step 10: Optional Decoration

• Add some fresh rosemary leaves on top to enhance the aroma.

Step 11: Enjoy this soup rich in mushrooms and aromas!

Pro Tip: Add a final touch with a drizzle of truffle oil before serving to intensify the flavors.

Green Lentil Broth with Turmeric

Ingredients:

• 1 cup of green lentils, washed • 1 chopped onion
• 2 chopped garlic
cloves • 1 sliced carrot

• 1 liter of vegetable broth • 1 teaspoon
of turmeric

• 1 tablespoon olive oil • Salt and pepper to taste

Method of preparation:

Step 1: Preparation of Ingredients

• Wash the green lentils under running water. • Chop the
onion, garlic cloves and cut the carrot into slices.

Step 2: Sautéing Aromatics

• Heat the olive oil in a large pan over medium heat. • Saute the onion and garlic until
golden and aromatic.

Step 3: Adding Lentils and Turmeric

• Add the green lentils and turmeric to the pan. Saute for a few minutes.

Step 4: Incorporating Broth

• Pour the liter of vegetable broth into the pan. Stir to incorporate the ingredients.

Step 5: Adding Carrot

• Add the carrot slices to the pan. Shake well.

Step 6: Seasoning

• Season with salt and pepper to taste. Stir again.

Step 7: Cooking

• Let the mixture boil. Reduce heat and simmer for 20-25 minutes, until lentils and carrots are tender.

Step 8: Adjusting the Flavor

• Taste and adjust seasoning if necessary.

Step 9: Serving

• Serve the Green Lentil Broth with Turmeric in individual bowls.

Step 10: Optional Decoration

• Add a touch of fresh parsley or coriander leaves on top.

Step 11: Enjoy this nutritious, spice-filled broth!

Pro Tip: Try drizzling with extra virgin olive oil when serving to enhance the flavors.

Tomato and Red Pepper Soup

Ingredients:

• 6 medium tomatoes, roasted • 2 red
peppers, roasted and skinless • 1 onion, chopped • 2 cloves
of garlic, chopped • 1
liter of vegetable broth • Fresh basil
leaves • 1 tablespoon of olive oil • Salt
and pepper August

Method of preparation:

Step 1: Preparation of Ingredients

• Roast the tomatoes and peppers in the oven until the skin is wrinkled. Peel the
  Bell peppers.
• Chop the onion and garlic cloves.

Step 2: Sautéing Aromatics

• Heat the olive oil in a large pan over medium heat. • Saute the onion and garlic until
golden and aromatic.

Step 3: Adding Tomatoes and Peppers

• Add the roasted tomatoes and skinless peppers to the pan. Sauté for a few
  minutes.

Step 4: Incorporating Broth

• Pour the liter of vegetable broth into the pan. Stir to incorporate the ingredients.

Step 5: Seasoning

• Season with salt and pepper to taste. Add basil leaves.

Step 6: Cooking

• Let the mixture boil. Reduce the heat and simmer for 15-20 minutes to release the
  flavors.

Step 7: Adjusting the Flavor

• Taste and adjust seasoning if necessary.

Step 8: Blending (Optional)

• Use an immersion blender to obtain a smoother consistency.

Step 9: Serving

• Serve the Tomato and Red Pepper Soup in individual bowls.

Step 10: Optional Decoration

• Add some fresh basil leaves on top.

Step 11: Enjoy this soup rich in toasty flavors and deliciously comforting!

Pro Tip: Serve with croutons or a sprinkle of Parmesan cheese.

Kale Soup with Chia

Ingredients:

• 1 bunch of kale, finely chopped • 1 onion,
chopped • 2 cloves of
garlic, chopped • 1 medium sweet
potato, cubed • 1 liter of vegetable broth • 2
tablespoons of chia seeds • 1
tablespoon of olive oil olive oil • Salt and pepper to taste

Method of preparation:

Step 1: Preparation of Ingredients

• Finely chop the cabbage, cut the onion into small pieces and the garlic cloves. • Cover the diced sweet
potatoes.

Step 2: Sautéing Aromatics

• Heat the olive oil in a large pan over medium heat. • Saute the onion and garlic until
golden and aromatic.

Step 3: Adding Kale and Sweet Potatoes

• Add the chopped kale and sweet potato to the pan. Saute for a few minutes.

Step 4: Incorporating Broth

• Pour the liter of vegetable broth into the pan. Stir to incorporate the ingredients.

Step 5: Adding Chia

• Add the chia seeds to the pan. Shake well.

Step 6: Seasoning

• Season with salt and pepper to taste. Stir again.

Step 7: Cooking

• Let the mixture boil. Reduce heat and simmer for 20-25 minutes, until sweet potatoes
become soft.

Step 8: Adjusting the Flavor

• Taste and adjust seasoning if necessary.

Step 9: Serving

• Serve Kale and Chia Soup in individual bowls.

Step 10: Optional Decoration

• Add a drizzle of olive oil or a touch of red pepper for extra flavor.

Step 11: Enjoy this nutritious soup full of textures!

Pro Tip: Serve with lemon wedges for a citrusy touch when serving.

Asparagus Cream with Basil

Ingredients:

• 500g fresh asparagus, lower part discarded • 1 chopped onion • 2
chopped garlic cloves •
1 diced potato

• 1 liter of vegetable broth • A handful
of fresh basil leaves • 1 tablespoon of olive oil • Salt and
pepper to taste

Method of preparation:

Step 1: Preparation of Ingredients

• Discard the lower part of the asparagus and cut the stalks into small pieces. • Chop the onion, garlic
cloves and potatoes.

Step 2: Sautéing Aromatics

• Heat the olive oil in a large pan over medium heat. • Saute the onion and garlic until
golden and aromatic.

Step 3: Adding Asparagus and Potatoes

• Add the asparagus and potatoes to the pan. Saute for a few minutes.

Step 4: Incorporating Broth

• Pour the liter of vegetable broth into the pan. Stir to incorporate the ingredients.

Step 5: Adding Basil

• Add the basil leaves to the pan. Shake well.

Step 6: Seasoning

• Season with salt and pepper to taste. Stir again.

Step 7: Cooking

• Let the mixture boil. Reduce the heat and simmer for 15-20 minutes, until the asparagus and
potatoes become soft.

Step 8: Adjusting the Flavor

• Taste and adjust seasoning if necessary.

Step 9: Liquidification

• Use an immersion blender to obtain a smooth cream.

Step 10: Serving

• Serve the Asparagus Cream with Basil in individual bowls.

Step 11: Optional Decoration

• Add some fresh basil leaves on top.

Step 12: Enjoy this delicate cream full of fresh flavors!

Pro Tip: Try drizzling with truffle oil or adding shavings of Parmesan before serving for an extra touch of sophistication.